INTERMITTENT FASTING FOR WOMEN OVER 50

NOT JUST THE GUIDE BUT THE ACTUAL PLAN WITH RECIPES TO LOSE WEIGHT, DETOX YOUR BODY AND ENHANCE LONGEVITY

only permitted with the publisher's express written consent. All other rights are reserved.

The material on the following pages is generally assumed to be a true and correct account of reality, and any inattention, use, or mis-use of the information by the reader would place any subsequent behavior solely under their control. There are no circumstances under which the publisher or the original author of this work may be held responsible for any suffering or damages that they may suffer as a consequence of using the information provided here.

Furthermore, the information on the following pages is provided solely for educational purposes and should not be considered universal. It is addressed without certainty as to its long-term validity or interim consistency, as befits its existence. The use of trademarks is achieved without written permission and should not be construed as an endorsement by the trademark holder.

TABLE OF CONTENT

CHAPTER 1

CHAPTER 2

INTRODUCTION

The world is full of diet fads. We had diet pills in the 1990s. You were missing out on life's quintessential health boosters if you didn't have a juicer in the early 1990s. Green tea pads that reduce tummy size have now been given to us, and if you don't eat like a Neanderthal, you're already at a disadvantage.

As a rule, I am skeptical of all fads. If something is marketed as revolutionary and game-changing in the world of weight loss, it's probably just marketing speak to sell whatever is currently popular. If there was ever a fad to get behind, it's intermittent fasting, and I'm so excited to share what I've learned about it with you.

When it comes to losing weight, women over 50 can have a difficult time. Variety of factors can cause this. The most common cause is a slowed metabolism. The faster your metabolism is, the leaner muscle you have. However, as we age, we lose lean muscle mass and become less active than we once were. What's the end result? Stubborn female body fat that refuses to go away.

Intermittent fasting has grown in popularity in recent years as a result of its numerous health benefits and the fact that it does not limit your food choices. Fasting has been shown to improve metabolism, mental health, and possibly helps some cancers, according to research. It can also protect women over 50 from certain muscle, nerve, and joint disorders.

Lower metabolism, achy joints, reduced muscle mass, and even sleep issues all make it more difficult to lose weight after 50. Simultaneously, losing fat, particularly dangerous belly fat, can significantly lower your risk of serious health problems like diabetes, heart attacks, and cancer.

Of course, as you get older, your chances of contracting a variety of health issue rises. When it comes to weight loss and reducing the risk of developing age-related illnesses, intermittent fasting for women over 50 may be a virtual fountain of youth in some cases.

Intermittent fasting, unlike most diets, focuses on when to eat by incorporating regular short-term fasts into your routine. This eating style may assist you in consuming fewer calories, losing weight, and reducing your risk of diabetes and heart problems.

Intermittent fasting, on the other hand, may not be as beneficial for women as it is for men, according to a number of studies. As a result, women may need to take a different approach.

Have you ever wondered how Jennifer Anniston stays in such good shape at her age as a woman in her fifties? "Intermittent Fasting" was the answer she gave in an interview. Many celebrities, including Kourtney Kardashian and Hugh Jackman, practice Intermittent Fasting because it is proven to be effective.

In 2020, one of the most popular searches on the internet was "intermittent fasting," and this diet continues to make headlines in 2021.

You've probably tried a number of diet plans to lose weight and get in shape, but they've only served to give you headaches and wreak havoc on your body. That's why, in order to heal your body and soul while losing weight, you'll need a scientifically proven method like intermittent fasting.

This book will teach you everything you need to know about Intermittent Fasting so you can begin your own healing and self-love journey.

History of Intermittent Fasting

Fasting is not a new notion. Humans have fasted for a variety of reasons, including overnight periods, religious reasons, and food scarcity. Fasting is thought to be one of the world's oldest healing practices. Fasting was recommended by Hippocrates of Cos, a Greek scientist. Fasting was also strongly advocated by other Greek scholars such as Plato and Aristotle.

Fasting was thought to be a universal tendency for a variety of ailments by the ancient Greeks. They also believed that it enhanced cognitive ability. Consider a day when your stomach was overflowing with food. Did you feel cognitively alert and energized afterward, or were you drowsy and sleepy?

Fasting is used to wash or purify the soul in various religions (including Islam, Christianity, and Buddhism). However, it effectively translates into the identical advantages that the Greek researchers have endorsed.

Modern intermittent fasting is all on gradually adopting fasting into your daily diet. It entails eating wisely most of the time and then going without food for an extended length of time every now and then. You can also have cheat days once a week, where you can overeat on a limited amount of food.

WHAT IS INTERMITTENT FASTING?

Intermittent fasting is a method of calorie restriction that involves a set of on and off periods of eating. I know it sounds boring and simple, but trust me, when I tried it, I quickly discovered that it is a self-discipline exercise that can be frustrating at first.

I've spent the majority of 2019 practicing intermittent fasting, and the results I've seen include weight loss, mental clarity, a full night's sleep, and a lot more energy. I began experimenting with intermittent fasting for the sake of longevity rather than weight loss. But the first thing I noticed was that my belly fat had significantly decreased.... Because you can't spot-reduce fat on your body, the loss of belly fat will have been due to hormones... and, as we all know, weight gain around the midsection is a fact of life during menopause.

Intermittent fasting is a tool that people I respect and follow in the field of longevity use to stay younger. Prof. David Sinclair of Harvard University, a longevity scientist and expert, made a statement that put my mind at ease... He claims that no one knows the exact answer or the ideal fasting method, even if they claim to.... Experiments on mice have shown that eating 30% less food increases lifespan by 30%.

What I liked about it was that it made intermittent fasting a little easier for me to follow because I knew it wasn't an exact science. You can become extremely stressed if you follow all of the experts and all of the small details involved. So, I'll tell you what I did, how I lost weight, and how I dealt with my hunger.

Fasting for 16-18 hours at a time has become increasingly popular in recent years. For the most part, this means waiting until noon to eat. Skipping dinner is less appealing because going to bed hungry contradicts one of the goals of IF, which is to increase Growth Hormone. The production of GH is reduced by tossing and turning due to hunger, with the greatest reduction occurring during deep sleep phases.

This contradicts the notion that the breakfast is the most important meal of the day as we believe. And it contradicts studies that show that eating the most protein first thing in the morning improves food choices throughout the day, if not fat metabolism.

Taking vitamins and drinking juices made from low-calorie vegetables is recommended during fasting periods. It maintains a consistent level of minerals and vitamins. Following the fasting window, there is an eating window. This window typically lasts 6 to 12 hours.

Because there are different IF methods, the fasting and eating windows can vary. Some IF methods are more intense than others. You can try out different methods to see which one works best for you and your lifestyle.

WHAT'S ALL THE FUSS ABOUT?

According to the most recent research on IF, this relatively simple dietary approach can help almost anything. Intermittent fasting will help you lose weight, gain muscle, raise your metabolism, lose fat, strengthen your memory, heal your body, and be more efficient, according to a sample of Amazon book titles.

Although all of these arguments would ring true for someone who has followed a fad diet, the science behind those bold book titles actually holds a lot of promise.

Experts warn, however, that there are risks involved. Fasting can be dangerous for people who have diabetes or other states that require them to keep their blood glucose levels stable. Low blood sugar can cause dizziness, lightheadedness, and confusion if you don't eat while you're exercising. Fasting can also cause dangerous electrolyte imbalances in people taking drugs for heart problems or high blood pressure.

There's also some science at work here, in the form of your body's HGH production. Before we get into that, let me explain why this is the case. Our bodies produce insulin to store glucose from carbohydrates for later use when we eat. We live in a society where most of our meals are routine, and we are constantly bombarded with foods that are high in sugar and fat. This puts us in an anabolic state, which means we're always gaining weight.

Food glucose is stored as fat, resulting in weight gain. Intermittent fasting effectively converse this process, allowing our cells to use the glucose that has been stored in our cells for energy. Weight loss occurs when cells enter a catabolic (breaking down) state. HGH is produced in response to your body's need for glucose, so when we eat frequently, our HGH production is suppressed because we are getting glucose from outside sources. HGH is a hormone that regulates metabolism and has numerous benefits for muscle repair and fat burning. Fasting for short periods of time has been shown to increase HGH production by up to 5 times.

Although further research is required to decide if and how IF and TRF can be most useful, researchers and other experts agree that it is already a valuable tool in the obesity battle. "Ultimately, the degree of dietary commitment and longevity, rather than the form of dietary plan, will predict weight-loss outcomes," as one study of the literature put it.

If you practice intermittent fasting, also known as IF, you won't have to starve yourself. It also doesn't give you permission to eat a lot of unhealthy food when you aren't fasting. Instead of eating meals and snacks throughout the day, you eat during a set period of time.

The majority of people adhere to an IF schedule that requires them to fast for 12 to 16 hours every day. They eat regular meals and snacks the rest of the time. Because most people sleep for about eight hours during their fasting hours, sticking to this eating window isn't as difficult as it sounds. You're also encouraged to drink zero-calorie beverages like water, tea, and coffee. Fast Bars can also be eaten in between meals to keep the fast going.

For the best intermittent fasting results, create an eating schedule that works for you. Consider the following example:

12-HOUR FASTS METHOD

You could skip breakfast and eat at lunch if you're on a 12-12 fast. You could eat an early supper and avoid evening snacks if you prefer to eat your morning meal. A 12-12 fast is relatively easy to maintain for most older women.

THE WARRIOR DIET

	DAY 1	DAY 2	DAY 3	DAY 4	DAY 5	DAY 6	DAY 7
Midnight 4 AM 8 AM 12 PM	Eating only small amounts of vegetables and fruits	Eating only small amounts of vegetables and fruits	Eating only small amounts of vegetables and fruits	Eating only small amounts of vegetables and fruits	Eating only small amounts of vegetables and fruits	Eating only small amounts of vegetables and fruits	Eating only small amounts of vegetables and fruits
4 PM	Large meal	Large meal	Large meal	Large meal	Large meal	Large meal	Large meal
8 PM Midnight							

16-HOUR FASTS METHOD:

A 16-8 IF schedule may help you achieve faster results. Within an 8-hour window, most people choose to eat two meals and a snack or two. For example, your eating window could be set between noon and 8 p.m., or between 8 a.m. and 4 p.m.

THE 16/8 METHOD

	DAY 1	DAY 2	DAY 3	DAY 4	DAY 5	DAY 6	DAY 7
Midnight / 4 AM / 8 AM	FAST	FAST	FAST	FAST	FAST	FAST	FAST
12 PM	First meal	First meal	First meal	First meal	First meal	First meal	First meal
4 PM	Last meal by 8pm	Last meal by 8pm	Last meal by 8pm	Last meal by 8pm	Last meal by 8pm	Last meal by 8pm	Last meal by 8pm
8 PM / Midnight	FAST	FAST	FAST	FAST	FAST	FAST	FAST

5:2 method:

Restricted eating periods may not be suitable for you on a daily basis. Another option is to follow a 12- or 16-hour fast for five days and then relax for two days. For example, you could do intermittent fasting during the week and eat normally on the weekends.

THE 5:2 DIET

DAY 1	DAY 2	DAY 3	DAY 4	DAY 5	DAY 6	DAY 7
Eats normally	Women: *500 calories* Men: *600 calories*	Eats normally	Eats normally	Women: *500 calories* Men: *600 calories*	Eats normally	Eats normally

ALTERNATE DAY METHOD:

You can eat normally every other day if you choose this method. On fasting days, you'll consume only 25% of your daily caloric requirements. For example, if you normally consume 1,800 calories per day, you will consume only 450 calories on fasting days.

ALTERNATE-DAY FASTING

DAY 1	DAY 2	DAY 3	DAY 4	DAY 5	DAY 6	DAY 7
Eats normally	24-hour fast OR Eat only a few hundred calories	Eats normally	24-hour fast OR Eat only a few hundred calories	Eats normally	24-hour fast OR Eat only a few hundred calories	Eats normally

24-HOUR METHOD:

Fasting for a full 24 hours before eating again is required for this method. Fasting from breakfast to breakfast or lunch to lunch is usually done once or twice a week by those who use this method.

EAT-STOP-EAT

DAY 1	DAY 2	DAY 3	DAY 4	DAY 5	DAY 6	DAY 7
Eats normally	24-hour fast	Eats normally	Eats normally	24-hour fast	Eats normally	Eats normally

SPONTANEOUS MEAL SKIPPING:

You don't have to stick to a strict intermittent fasting schedule to reap any of the benefits. Another choice is to miss meals on occasion, such as when you aren't hungry or when you are too busy to prepare and eat.

It's a misconception that people must eat every few hours or risk malnutrition or muscle loss. Your body is designed to withstand long stretches of hunger, let alone missing one or two meals every now and then.

SPONTANEOUS MEAL SKIPPING

DAY 1	DAY 2	DAY 3	DAY 4	DAY 5	DAY 6	DAY 7
Breakfast	Skipped Meal	Breakfast	Breakfast	Breakfast	Breakfast	Breakfast
Lunch	Lunch	Lunch	Lunch	Lunch	Lunch	Lunch
Dinner	Dinner	Dinner	Dinner	Skipped Meal	Dinner	Dinner

EVERY-OTHER-DAY FASTS METHOD: On alternate days, another variation calls for severely calorie-restricted eating. For instance, you could restrict your calories to under 500 calories one day and then eat normally the next. It's worth noting that daily IF fasts never necessitate calorie restrictions that low.

You'll get the best results from this diet if you stick to it. At the same time, on special occasions, you can certainly take a break from this type of eating schedule. You should try different types of intermittent fasting to see which one works best for you. Many people begin their IF journey with the 12-12 plan and then progress to the 16-8 plan. After that, try to stick to your plan as closely as possible.

WHAT MAKES INTERMITTENT FASTING WORK?

Some people believe that IF has helped them lose weight simply because the limited eating window forces them to eat fewer calories. For example, instead of three meals and two snacks, they may only have time for two meals and one snack. They become more conscious of the foods they eat and tend to avoid processed carbohydrates, unhealthy fats, and empty calories.

Of course, you have the freedom to eat whatever healthy foods you want. While some people use intermittent fasting to reduce their overall calorie intake, others use it in conjunction with a keto, vegan, or other diet.

Intermittent fasting helps you eat less calories, which is why it helps you lose weight. During the fasting periods, all of the procedures require skipping meals. You will consume less calories unless you compensate by eating substantially more during the meal hours.

Intermittent fasting reduced body weight by 3–8% over a period of 3–24 weeks, according to a 2014 review. When it comes to weight loss, intermittent fasting has been shown to generate weight reduction of 0.55 to 1.65 pounds (0.25–0.75 kg) every week. The waist circumference of the participants decreased by 4–7%, indicating that they shed belly fat.

These findings suggest that intermittent fasting could be an effective weight-loss strategy.

However, the advantages of intermittent fasting extend far beyond weight loss. It also has several metabolic health benefits and may possibly help lower the risk of cardiovascular disease. Although calorie counting is not necessary when conducting intermittent fasting, the weight loss is mostly mediated by a reduction in overall calorie consumption.

When calories are matched between groups, studies comparing intermittent fasting and continuous calorie restriction indicate no difference in weight loss.

While there are distinct guidelines for different types of fasting, intermittent fasts generally follow the same basic principles: Limit your calorie consumption during certain times of the day and eat normally at others. This diet, like any other, lowers your overall calorie intake, but it also helps you lose weight in another way.

Here's how it works: You obtain energy from the glucose (sugar) in your meal whenever you eat. Insulin, a hormone generated by the pancreas, aids glucose delivery to the body's cells. There, glucose is either used for energy right away or stored for later use.

When you don't eat carbohydrates or any other source of energy, your body automatically suppresses insulin production. If your insulin levels go low enough, your body will use the glucose stored in your cells as a source of energy. When those are gone, it turns to fat for sustenance. This aids with weight loss.

And many people lose weight on IF, at least in the beginning. However, the average weight loss is modest, and as with all diets, the weight usually returns once the diet is over. Over the course of 24 weeks, participants in a 2018 meta-analysis dropped only 0.38 percent of their body weight on average. Another randomized controlled research published the same year indicated that people who were overweight or obese lost 7.1 percent in 12 weeks on IF, but gained nearly 2 percent back 9 months later.

The actual causes of ageing are unknown, however metabolic rates and free radicals appear to play a role in the ageing process regardless of whether either of these theories is totally correct.

Calorie restriction comes into play because it is well known that dramatically lowering food intake lowers metabolic rate. If less food is consumed, the body will have less food to metabolize. Furthermore, because calorie restriction usually leads to weight reduction, less energy is required to sustain the lower body mass.

Calorie restriction is thought to extend lifespans through lowering the rate of free radical damage as a result of this reduced metabolic rate. This theory is backed up by actual evidence that some animals release fewer free radicals when they are deprived of calories. Although there is no consensus on the optimal approach to assess free radical damage specifically, there is some evidence that calorie restriction can reduce protein and DNA damage. This shows that restricting calories slows the ageing process, allowing an organism to live longer and with a lower risk of age-related disorders.

HEALTH BENEFITS OF INTERMITTENT FASTING FOR WOMEN

While some nutritionists believe that IF (Intermittent Fasting) only works because it encourages people to eat less, others disagree. They believe that with the same number of calories and other nutrients, intermittent fasting produces better results than traditional meal schedules. Studies have even suggested that fasting for several hours a day accomplishes more than just calorie restriction.

"Fasting causes glucose [blood sugar] levels to drop. After converting fat into ketones, the body uses fat instead of glucose as a source of energy "Kathy McManus, director of the Department of Nutrition at the Harvard-affiliated Brigham and Women's Hospital, explains. The switch from glucose to ketones as a source of energy has a positive impact on body chemistry.

Animals who fast regularly lose weight, have lower blood pressure and heart rates, have less insulin resistance, have lower "bad" LDL cholesterol levels, higher "good" HDL cholesterol levels, and have less inflammation. Improved memory has also been discovered in some studies.

At least in animals, intermittent fasting is linked to a longer lifespan. What is the reason for this? Intermittent fasting, according to recent Harvard research, may allow each cell's energy-producing engines (mitochondria) to produce energy more efficiently and maintain a more youthful state.

Intermittent fasting can help you lose weight while also lowering your risk of developing a variety of chronic problems.

IS INTERMITTENT FASTING HEALTHY?

Is intermittent fasting a healthy way to eat? Remember that you should only fast for 12 to 16 hours at a time, not for days. You still have plenty of time to eat a delicious and healthy meal. Of course, some older women may require frequent eating due to metabolic disorders or prescription instructions. In that case, you should talk to your doctor about your eating habits before making any changes.

While it isn't technically fasting, some doctors claim that allowing easy-to-digest foods like whole fruit during the fasting window has health benefits. Modifications like these can still provide a much-needed break for your digestive and metabolic systems. For example, the popular weight-loss book "Fit for Life" recommended eating only fruit after supper and before lunch.

In reality, research on patients who only changed their eating habits by fasting for 12 to 16 hours per day. Despite not adhering to the diet's other guidelines or counting calories, they lost weight and improved their health. This technique may have succeeded precisely because dieters swapped fast food for whole foods. In either case, participants considered this dietary adjustment to be beneficial and simple to implement. Traditionalists won't call this fasting, but it's good to realize that you have choices if you can't go without food for more than a few hours.

It's not easy to adjust to intermittent fasting, especially if you're doing it all at once. One thing we must absolutely avoid during our eating periods is bingeing on large amounts of processed foods. We might not see any results if we do this! First and foremost, I recommend that you change your eating habits. Before attempting intermittent fasting, getting into a routine of eating as healthily as possible will be extremely beneficial. Start doing this two weeks before you plan to start your intermittent fasting schedule, and it will make the transition much easier.

It's difficult to stay on track, but here's what I did to stay on track.

1. I made a point of not snacking at night. This was by far the most difficult task for me, and it was where I expended the majority of my energy. But I remembered what David Sinclair said about hunger being a reminder of the good you're doing to your body during the day. As a result, I trained my mind to accept those minor hunger pangs throughout the day. I know I'll be able to eat soon, and I'm doing my part to improve my overall health.

2. I used Himalayan rock salt to deceive my body into thinking it wasn't hungry. When I'm hungry, I put a couple of granules under my tongue and forget that

I'm hungry. When I first heard about this, I had no idea it would work, but it does!

3. I read that when you're fasting, you shouldn't take any supplements because your body needs to do all the work on its own. So that's what I did, and it seems to be working well for me.
4. If I'm having a particularly hectic day, I'll do a 20/4 fast so that I don't have to worry about food, meal preparation, or planning. Depending on what I'm doing, I switch up my fasting times. But I always return to the fast because it makes me feel fantastic.
5. When I break my fast, the first thing I eat is protein. It has nothing to do with fat or carbohydrates. That has a positive effect on my body.

WHY FAST?

Humans have practiced fasting for thousands of years. When there was absolutely no food available, it was sometimes done out of desperation. It was also done for religious purposes in some cases. Fasting is required by many religions, including Islam, Christianity, and Buddhism. When humans and other animals are sick, they often react quickly.

Fasting is clearly not "unnatural," and our bodies are perfectly capable of going without food for long periods of time. When we don't eat for a while, our bodies go through a variety of changes in order to help us to survive during a famine. Hormones, chromosomes, and crucial cellular repair processes are all involved.

When we fast, our blood sugar and insulin levels drop significantly, while our levels of human growth hormone skyrocket. Many people use intermittent fasting to lose weight because it is a quick and easy way to cut calories and burn fat.

Others do so to increase their metabolic health, which can improve a variety of risk factors and health markers. Intermittent fasting has also been shown to help people live longer. It can prolong lifespan as effectively as calorie restriction in rodents, according to studies.

It can also help protect against problems such as heart health, type 2 diabetes, cancer, Alzheimer's, and others, according to some studies. Others prefer intermittent fasting because it is more convenient.

It's a useful "life hack" that helps you simplify your life while also improving your health. Your life would be easier if you just have to prepare a few meals. It also saves time not having to eat 3-4 times a day with all the planning and cleaning that entails.

TAKE HOME MESSAGE

Restricting you're eating window and fasting on occasion can have some very impressive health benefits as long as you stick to nutritious foods. It's an efficient way to lose weight and improve metabolic health while also simplifying your life.

Consider occasions when you go without food for extended periods of time. Ask yourself the following questions if you're actually experimenting with intermittent fasting (whether knowingly or because your dieting attitude has crept into your food control):

- Do you feel like you're getting weaker or having less stamina?
- Have you found that the same exercises are becoming more difficult?
- Is the consistency of your sleep deteriorating?
- Do you have any trouble concentrating or focusing?
- Do you find yourself being more nervous, frustrated, or forgetful?
- Is hunger causing you to become distracted?

If you answered yes to all of these questions, IF is probably not for you at this time.

WOMEN AND INTERMITTENT FASTING

If you're a female with fluctuating hormones or high levels of perceived stress (all that counts is how much stress you feel), IF may be another stressor that raises cortisol levels or causes them to crash even further if you have adrenal fatigue. That is, you've been under a lot of stress for a long time and haven't been able to balance it out with coping strategies due to poor diet or other lifestyle habits. Your body will eventually run out of cortisol to produce. To control life, we need it at appropriate levels.

When you purposefully add a stressor for some reason, the trick is to momentarily delete it somewhere else. That isn't usually the case when someone chooses IF. How do you juggle work and home life stressors while maintaining a high-intensity workout routine? That's a very one-sided and unbalanced scale.

Take, for example, our Olympic athletes. The majority of them train as a career. They remain in Rio's athlete's quarters and eat meals made for athletes. They are completely focused on the minutes, if not seconds, that they will perform. They teach their brains to stop multitasking in order to reduce tension. Their best results are the product of their greatest concentration. It's the same for your body. When dietary and exercise stressors are added to already existing stressors, the outcome can be the polar opposite of what you want.

WOMEN VERSUS MEN

On ADF (alternate daily fasting), both men and women experienced substantial reductions in insulin, ketones (beta-hydroxy butyrate), and free fatty acids, indicating that both men and women would benefit. While the women had higher levels of hunger hormones, this finding was not shown in all tests.

Following three weeks of alternate day fasting, women were less effective at clearing glucose after a meal, according to a separate study on the same group of fasters. It's worth noting that this improvement was only observed in women; men's glucose clearance remained unchanged. What does this imply for females? It's difficult to extrapolate these findings since the participants were told they should consume twice as much on their eating days, which is unusual.

SHOULD WOMEN OVER 40 DO INTERMITTENT FASTING?

For women over 40, I believe intermittent fasting is a healthy choice. Several studies involving women over the age of 40 have shown that these diets are a healthy and safe choice. If you have type 2 diabetes or another health problem that necessitates a therapeutic diet, I recommend consulting with a registered dietitian. For many people, intermittent fasting (IF) is a more sustainable alternative to the conventional approach to continuous calorie restriction.

WHAT HAPPENS TO YOUR BODY IF YOU OVER-EAT?

No, your stomach is not going to burst. Continue reading to learn what happens to the body after a very large meal.

You already have a good idea of what happens if you consume too much food over time. But what if you eat too much at dinner? There are some things going on in your body besides being fully packed. We spoke with two dietitians to learn more about what happens to your metabolism and body when you consume too much. Also included are suggestions for what to do if you're feeling bloated.

WHAT HAPPENS AFTER A BIG MEAL?

When you eat, the stomach expands to accommodate the amount of food you've eaten. The brain receives signals from a stretched or full stomach that you are full. When you eat too much, your stomach expands beyond its usual size, leaving you feeling bloated. When the contents of the stomach move into the small intestine, this may cause pressure and discomfort.

"An extra-large meal can cause intestinal distress and probably acid reflux, which can be very uncomfortable in the short term." Acid reflux is a state in which stomach acid backs up into the esophagus, causing a bitter taste or burning sensation. This is particularly troublesome if the meal is eaten close to bedtime, as lying down can exacerbate the effects and disrupt sleep.

Blood sugar levels can also rise, particularly if you consume a lot of carbohydrates. After a meal, blood sugar (glucose) increases, but refined carbohydrates spike it the most, compared to high-fiber carbs or carbs with protein and fat. As blood sugar levels increase, the pancreas secretes the hormone insulin, which transports glucose from the bloodstream to the cells, where it is used for energy. Extra glucose is processed in the liver and muscles as glycogen. Any excess glucose is then processed as fat.

WHAT HAPPENS IF YOU EAT TOO MUCH OVER TIME?

"In the long run, consuming more calories than you consume will lead to weight gain," says Harris-Pincus. "It can also cause a spike in blood sugar, especially if the larger meals are high in refined carbohydrates and sugar."

Overeating, also in the short term, has been shown to induce insulin resistance, in which cells refuse to take up the glucose that insulin is attempting to deliver. As a result, blood sugar levels remain high, which can lead to obesity and type 2 diabetes over time. In a 2017 report, young, healthy adults with one day of binge eating had decreased blood sugar regulation and insulin sensitivity.

Leptin resistance can also be caused by eating too much over time. Leptin is a hormone released by fat cells that tells the brain when it's time to eat. The higher a person's body fat percentage is, the more leptin they produce.

Leptin resistance, on the other hand, occurs when the brain does not receive the signal from leptin to avoid feeding. As a result, appetite remains high, leading to a vicious cycle of overeating, which can lead to additional fat gain. Triglyceride levels can also be raised by overeating, particularly if you eat too many high-sugar foods or drink too much alcohol.

When it comes to your stomach, ""A single large meal, such as Thanksgiving dinner, will not cause your stomach to 'stretch' [permanently] because it is designed to expand and contract to satisfy your normal food intake," Harris-Pincus explains, but "consistently eating beyond when you are full will cause your stomach to expand to manage the chronic extra food." To be happy on a regular basis, you will need to consume more food. To stop overeating, the only way to avoid it is to pay attention to the body's appetite and fullness signals."

WHAT DO YOU DO IF YOU'VE OVER-EATEN?

First and foremost, Manaker advises, "don't be too hard on yourself." What you do most of the time is more important than what you do sometimes. "You should chew ginger, drink ginger tea, or take black licorice root to get some immediate relief. Taking a stroll may also provide some relaxation. Maintaining an upright posture and avoiding lying down will also help to reduce the risk of heartburn. Avoid carbonated drinks and instead opt for flat water "she explains.

"Pay attention to whether something is causing this behavior if you find yourself consistently overeating," Manaker advises. Are you eating because you're mentally hungry or because you're stressed? Many people, whether deliberately or accidentally, overeat in the evening because they didn't eat enough throughout the day. At each meal, aim for protein, fiber, and healthy fats, and eat every 3-4 hours.

Arrive at meals hungry but not famished. If you arrive hungry, you are more likely to eat quickly and then overeat because your stomach does not have time to signal your brain that you are full. Since your blood sugar has dropped so low, your body craves the quickest source of energy—sugar—you're more likely to search for easy carbohydrates first. To help you measure hunger and fullness during the day, use a hunger scale of 1-10 that ranges from not hungry to stuffed. Slow down when eating and try to finish a meal in 20 minutes.

"Keeping track of your portions will help you avoid repeating this action. Having a snack before a meal, such as a handful of nuts, will make you feel less hungry at mealtime and possibly control your portion sizes."

MY NOTES ON INTERMITTENT FASTING

Intermittent fasting has totally reframed a significant part of my knowledge of healthy eating habits and opened up a whole new world of healthy ageing and longevity for me. I would love for all of you to give it a shot, and I'll lay out my thoughts and recommendations for getting started.

As a disclaimer, I am not a healthcare professional, and before attempting this on your own, I recommend consulting with a healthcare professional to determine if it is appropriate for you.

The act of restricting calories is a catalyst for weight loss in and of itself, so that seems like a no-brainer.

A 12-hour fast would be an excellent place to start your intermittent fasting journey. You'll have started your intermittent fasting journey if you finish your last meal by 8 p.m. and don't eat again until 8 a.m. the next day. The 12-hour fast will assist you in establishing a positive mindset and developing the discipline necessary to establish a regular eating pattern.

When you're used to fasting for 12 hours... Experiment with waiting until noon before eating your first meal. If you succeed, your body will have been fasting for 16 hours. The next step is to fast for another 4 hours and only eat between 2pm and 6pm. I recommend trying different things to see what works best for your body. I wouldn't recommend attempting a 20-hour fast until you've properly prepared your body, but it's certainly a goal you can set for yourself if you want to lose more weight and feel fantastic.... Note: You can fast every other day if you want don't stress, you don't have to get it perfect!

If you can make it until noon. You've skipped one meal of the day, which equates to 30% less food (technically). Weight loss is achieved by eating less and exercising more, but here's what I like about it: animal tests revealed that when mice overate outside of fasting times, their lifespan was still increased by 30%, implying that it's not so much what you eat as it is when you eat. I strongly advise you to eat.

CHAPTER 2

PROS AND CONS OF INTERMITTENT FASTING

ntermittent fasting (IF) has been used to treat a variety of ailments for ages.

There are many various types of IF, ranging from plans that remove meals entirely on certain days to regimens that restrict eating just at particular times of the day. Different eating patterns have gotten a lot of attention as a means to achieve and maintain a healthy weight and obtain wellness benefits even in people who are already healthy.

The benefits and drawbacks of intermittent fasting are still being studied. Long-term studies are needed to determine whether this eating regimen produces long-term benefits.

PROS

- Easy to follow
- There will be no calorie counting
- There are no restrictions on macronutrients
- There are no restrictions on what you can eat
- Longevity may be improved
- Helps you lose weight
- Glucose management may be improved
- Other health advantages are possible

- Fasting-related side effects on days you are fasting
- It's possible that it'll make you feel a lot less active
- Concerns for folks who are taking prescription drugs
- Doesn't promote healthy eating habits
- It's possible that it'll encourage you to eat too much.
- It's also possible that it won't be good for you in the long term

PROS - EXPLAINED

EASY TO FOLLOW

Many dietary plans emphasize eating some foods while limiting or avoiding others. Learning the exact principles of an eating style can take a significant amount of time. There are entire books dedicated to learning how to understand the DASH diet or how to follow a Mediterranean-style food plan, for example.

THERE WILL BE NO CALORIE COUNTING

People who are attempting to achieve or maintain a healthy weight, predictably, prefer to avoid calorie counting. While many goods include nutrition labels, the process of estimating portion sizes and tabulating daily counts, whether manually or through a smartphone app, can be time consuming.

People are more likely to stick to regimens when all pre-measured calorie-controlled items are available, according to a 2011 study. However, many people do not have the financial means to pay for such programs, especially in the long run.

THERE ARE NO RESTRICTIONS ON MACRONUTRIENTS

There are a number of popular diet programs that severely limit specific macronutrients. Many people, for example, follow a low-carb diet to improve their health or lose weight. Others eat a low-fat diet for medical reasons or to lose weight.

Each of these programs demands the client to adopt a new eating pattern, typically substituting new and possibly unfamiliar items for old favorites. This may necessitate learning new culinary techniques as well as learning to shop and equip the kitchen in a new way.

Because there is no target macronutrient range and no macronutrient is limited or disallowed, none of these abilities are necessary when intermittent fasting.

NO RESTRICTIONS ON WHAT YOU CAN EAT

Anyone who has ever adjusted their diet for medical reasons or to achieve a healthy weight understands that you begin to crave items that you are not supposed to eat.

In fact, a 2017 study found that an increased desire to eat is a primary cause to failed weight loss attempts.

However, on an intermittent fasting schedule, this issue is much reduced. Food restriction happens only during specific hours, and you can eat whatever you want during the plan's non-fasting hours or days. In fact, these days are commonly referred to as "feasting" days by scholars.

Of course, continuing to eat harmful foods may not be the healthiest approach to reap the benefits of intermittent fasting, but eliminating them on certain days reduces your overall intake and may give benefits in the long run.

LONGEVITY MAY BE IMPROVED

Longevity is one of the most often touted advantages of intermittent fasting. Rodent studies, according to the National Institute on Aging, have demonstrated that when mice are put on regimens that severely restrict calories (typically during fasting times), many of them live longer and have fewer diseases, including malignancies.

Is this advantage also available to humans? It does, according to those who promote the diets. Long-term research, however, are required to validate the advantage. There has been observational studies correlating religious fasting to long-term longevity benefits, according to a review published in 2010, although it was difficult to identify if fasting caused the benefit or if other factors played a role.

PROMOTES WEIGHT LOSS

The authors of a review of intermittent fasting study published in 2018 say that the studies they looked at indicated a significant reduction in fat mass among clinical trial participants. They also discovered that intermittent fasting, regardless of body mass index, was effective in weight loss. Longer-term research are needed, according to the article, despite the fact that short-term weight loss was examined.

In a major meta-analysis published in 2018, researchers looked at the results of 11 trials that lasted between 8 and 24 weeks. When it came to weight loss and metabolic improvements, the authors of the study concluded that both intermittent fasting and constant energy restriction had equivalent outcomes. Longer-term experiments, they said, are needed to make definitive conclusions.

It's also probable that weight loss outcomes are influenced by age. The effects of intermittent fasting (time-restricted feeding) on young (20-year-old) versus older (50-year-old) males were investigated in a study published in the journal Nutrition in 2018. Intermittent fasting reduced body mass modestly in young men but not in older individuals. Muscle power, on the other hand, was similar in both groups.

In 2018, some intermittent fasting studies suggested that while this eating style may assist people with type 2 diabetes regulate their blood sugar levels by causing weight reduction in overweight or obese people, it may also reduce insulin sensitivity in healthy people.

Fasting (together with medical supervision and 6-hour long dietary training) was shown to be beneficial in reversing insulin resistance while maintaining blood sugar management over a 7-month period in a case series reported in 2018. In these three cases, patients were able to quit taking insulin, lose weight, shrink their waist circumference, and improve their blood glucose levels overall.

However, with a bigger sample size and constant medical advice, another study published in 2019 found a less striking impact on blood glucose control. In adults with type 2 diabetes, researchers conducted a 24-month follow-up of a 12-month study comparing intermittent fasting with continuous calorie restriction. At 24 months, HbA1c levels increased in both the constant and intermittent calorie restriction groups.

These findings were in line with those of earlier research, which showed that blood glucose levels in people with type 2 diabetes can rise over time despite a variety of dietary treatments. The authors of the study do say that intermittent energy restriction may be better than continuous caloric restriction for sustaining lower HbA1c levels, but that more research with bigger sample sizes is needed to validate this.

SIDE EFFECTS

Certain negative effects may arise during the fasting period of the eating regimen, according to studies looking into the benefits of intermittent fasting.

Feeling moody, fatigued, experiencing exhaustion, heartburn, constipation, dehydration, poor sleep quality, or anemia are all common symptoms. Intermittent fasting may be harmful if you have hypertension, high LDL cholesterol, excessively high uric acid levels in the blood, hyperglycemia, cardiovascular disease, or liver and kidney illness.

REDUCED PHYSICAL ACTIVITY

The lack in physical activity may be one of the most noticeable negative effects of intermittent fasting. The majority of intermittent fasting programs do not include a physical activity recommendation. Unsurprisingly, people who adhere to the plans may become so exhausted that they fail to fulfil their daily step objectives and may even abandon their normal exercise routines.

It's been suggested that more research be done to see how intermittent fasting affects physical activity habits.

In the fasting stage of an IF eating plan, it's not uncommon for people to feel extremely hungry. When they are around individuals who are eating regular meals and snacks, their hunger may become more intense.

PEOPLE TAKING MEDICATIONS

Many people who take drugs find that taking them with meal alleviates some of the negative side effects. Some medications, in fact, specifically state that they should be taken with food. As a result, taking drugs while fasting may be difficult.

Before beginning an IF protocol, anyone who takes medication should consult with their doctor to ensure that the fasting stage will not interfere with the medicine's effectiveness or negative effects.

NO FOCUS ON NUTRITIOUS EATING

Most intermittent fasting programs focus on timing rather than food selection. As a result, no foods are avoided (including those that are low in nutrition), and those that are high in nutrition are not promoted. As a result, those who adhere to the diet are unlikely to learn how to consume a nutritious diet.

It's unlikely that you'll learn basic healthy eating and cooking skills, such as how to cook with healthy oils, eat more veggies, and choose whole grains over refined grains, if you're on a short-term intermittent fasting program for weight reduction or medical reasons.

INTERMITTENT FASTING MAY PROMOTE OVEREATING

Meal quantity and frequency are not restricted during the "feasting" stage of many intermittent fasting methods. Instead, customers can eat as much as they want. Unfortunately, this may encourage some people to overeat. If you feel starved after a day of complete fasting, for example, you may be tempted to overeat (or eat the wrong things) on days when "feasting" is permitted.

LONG-TERM LIMITATIONS

While intermittent fasting is not a new practice, much of the research into the benefits of this eating strategy is. As a result, it's difficult to say if the benefits will last. Furthermore, researchers frequently state that long-term studies are required to ascertain whether the eating plan is safe for more than a few months.

For the time being, the safest course of action is to choose and begin an IF program in consultation with your healthcare provider. To ensure that the eating pattern is beneficial for you, your health care team can track your progress, including health advantages and concerns.

CHAPTER 3

DELICIOUS RECIPES

You'll need substantial go-to meals that will keep you full all day, if you're eating within a twelve-hour, eight-hour, or four-hour span! If you're considering a high-protein diet for that purpose, you'll find all of the information you need right here.

SPICY CHOCOLATE KETO FAT BOMBS

INGREDIENTS

- 2/3 cup coconut oil
- 2/3 cup smooth peanut butter
- 1/2 cup dark cocoa
- 4 (6 g) packets stevia (or to taste)
- 1 tablespoon ground cinnamon
- 1/4 teaspoon kosher salt
- 1/2 cup toasted coconut flakes
- 1/4 teaspoon cayenne (to taste)

DIRECTIONS:

In a double boiler set over a pot of simmering water, combine coconut oil, peanut butter, and cocoa powder. Heat and whisking constantly, until you see the chocolate is melted and smooth. Stir in the stevia, cinnamon, and salt until all is well combined.

Fill a silicone mini muffin tray halfway with the mixture. (Alternatively, divide the mixture among the liners in a mini muffin tin lined with liners.)

Iranster to the treezer for 30 minutes to firm up the coconut and cayenne.

MILLET & QUINOA MEDITERRANEAN SALAD

INGREDIENTS

- 1⁄2 cup millet
- 1 cup water
- 1⁄2 cup quinoa (red, white, or black)
- 3⁄4 cup water
- 1 English cucumber, diced
- 1 tomatoes, ripe, seeds squeezed out, diced
- 1 sweet pepper, seeded, diced
- 1⁄2 red onion, sliced thin
- 1 garlic clove, pressed
- 200g feta cheese, diced
- 1 (10 ounce) can large white beans, drained
- 1⁄4 teaspoon cayenne pepper (more, to taste)
- 2 teaspoons dried dill (sub basil or oregano, if preferred)
- 1⁄4 cup pine nuts
- 1 lemon, juice of (zest as well, if preferred)
- 1 tablespoon olive oil (optional)
- fresh ground pepper, to taste

DIRECTIONS

Bring millet and 1 cup water to a boil, then reduce to a low heat and continue to cook for five minutes. Take the pan off the oven, cover it, and set it aside for ten minutes.

Bring quinoa and 3/4 cup water to a boil, then reduce to a low heat and cover and cook for 12-14 minutes, fluffing occasionally.

Toss all of the ingredients together and relax. Have fun!

FRENCH VANILLA ALMOND GRANOLA

INGREDIENTS

- 3 1/2 cups old fashioned oats (not quick)
- 1/2 cup sliced almonds
- 1/2 cup water
- 1/2 cup natural cane sugar
- 1/4 teaspoon salt
- 1/4 cup organic canola oil or 1/4 cup grapeseed oil
- 1 tablespoon vanilla extract

DIRECTIONS

Preheat the oven to 200 degrees Fahrenheit. Using parchment paper, line a big, rimmed cookie sheet.

Combine the oats and almonds in a big mixing bowl.

Stir the sugar and salt into the water in a small saucepan over medium heat. Cook, while stirring constantly, until the sugar has dissolved completely. Remove the pan from the sun. Combine the canola oil and vanilla extract in a mixing bowl. Stir in the oat and almond mixture until it is well mixed.

Bake for 2 hours, or until mixture is dry to the touch, on a lined cookie sheet. Stirring is not allowed! Remove from the oven and set aside to cool before slicing into chunks. Keep the jar airtight.

POACHED EGGS & AVOCADO TOASTS

INGREDIENTS

- 4 eggs
- 2 ripe avocados
- 2 teaspoons lemon juice (or juice of 1 lime)
- 4 slices thick bread
- 1 cup cheese (grated, edam, gruyere or whatever you have on hand)
- salt & freshly ground black pepper
- 4 teaspoons butter (for spreading on toast)

DIRECTIONS

Use your preferred tool to poach eggs.

Meanwhile, strip the stones from the avocados and cut them in half.

Scoop the flesh into a bowl with a spoon, then add the lemon or lime juice, salt, and pepper.

Using a fork, mash the potatoes roughly.

Butter the toast and spread it with butter.

Top each slice of buttered toast with the avocado mixture and a poached egg.

Serve immediately with a grating cheese sprinkle on top.

With fresh or grilled tomato halves on the side, these are both delicious.

SWEET POTATO CURRY WITH SPINACH AND CHICKPEAS

INGREDIENTS

- 1/2 large sweet onions, chopped or 2 scallions, thinly sliced
- 1 -2 teaspoon canola oil
- 2 tablespoons curry powder
- 1 tablespoon cumin
- 1 teaspoon cinnamon
- 10 ounces fresh spinach, washed, stemmed and coarsely chopped
- 2 large sweet potatoes, peeled and diced (about 2 lbs)
- 1 (14 1/2 ounce) can chickpeas, rinsed and drained
- 1/2 cup water
- 1 (14 1/2 ounce) can diced tomatoes, can substitute fresh if available
- 1/4 cup chopped fresh cilantro, for garnish
- basmati rice or brown rice, for serving

DIRECTIONS

You can cook the sweet potatoes in any way you like.

I peel, chop, and steam mine for about 15 minutes in a veggie steamer. Baking or boiling are also viable options.

Heat 1-2 tsp canola or vegetable oil over medium heat when sweet potatoes are cooking.

Add the onions and cook for 2-3 minutes, or until they soften.

Stir in the curry powder, cumin, and cinnamon to uniformly cover the onions in spices.

Stir in the tomatoes and their juices, as well as the chickpeas.

Increase the heat to a deep simmer for about a minute or two after adding 12 cup water.

Then, a few handfuls at a time, apply the fresh spinach, stirring to cover with the cooking liquid.

When all of the spinach has been added to the pan, cover and cook for 3 minutes, or until just wilted.

Stir the cooked sweet potatoes into the liquid to coat them.

Cook for another 3-5 minutes, or until all of the flavours are well blended.

Serve immediately after transferring to a serving dish and tossing with fresh cilantro.

This dish goes well with basmati or brown rice.

PEACH BERRY SMOOTHIE

INGREDIENTS

- 1 cup frozen peaches
- 1/4 cup coconut milk (adjust for thicker or thinner smoothie)
- 1/2 cup Greek yogurt
- 1/2 teaspoon almond flavoring

DIRECTIONS

In a high-powered blender, combine peaches and almond flavoring.

Check the thickness and make any necessary adjustments. If you want it thinner, add more milk, and if you want it thicker, add more peaches.

Chia seeds, berries, and slivered almonds are lovely additions.

Enjoy!

CROCK POT BLACK EYED PEAS

INGREDIENTS

- 1 (16 ounce) bag dried black-eyed peas
- 1 small ham hock
- 1 (14 1/2 ounce) can Del Monte zesty jalapeno pepper diced tomato
- 1 (14 1/2 ounce) can diced tomatoes with green chilies
- 2 (10 1/2 ounce) cans chicken broth
- 1 stalk celery, chopped

DIRECTIONS

Soak the black-eyed peas as directed on the box.

Combine all ingredients in a slow cooker and steam for 9-10 hours on medium.

SWEET POTATO AND BLACK BEAN BURRITO

INGREDIENTS:

- 5cups peeled cubed sweet potatoes
- 1/2 teaspoon salt
- 2 (2) teaspoons other vegetable oil or 2 teaspoons broth
- 3 1/2 cups diced onions
- 4 garlic cloves, minced (or pressed)
- 1 tablespoon minced fresh green chili pepper
- 4 teaspoons ground cumin
- 4 teaspoons ground coriander
- 4 1/2 cups cooked black beans (three 15-ounce cans, drained)
- 2/3 cup lightly packed cilantro leaf
- 2 tablespoons fresh lemon juice
- 1 teaspoon salt
- 12 (10 inch) flour tortillas

DIRECTIONS:

Preheat the oven to 350 degrees Fahrenheit.

In a medium saucepan, combine the sweet potatoes, salt, and enough water to cover them.

Cover and bring to a boil, then reduce to a low heat and cook until the vegetables are tender, about 10 minutes.

Drain the water and set it aside.

Heat the oil in a medium skillet or saucepan and add the onions, garlic, and chile while the sweet potatoes are cooking.

Cover and cook on medium-low heat, stirring periodically, for around 7 minutes, or until the onions are tender.

Cook, stirring regularly, for another 2 to 3 minutes after adding the cumin and coriander.

Place the pan to the side after removing it from the fire.

In a food processor, puree the black beans, cilantro, lemon juice, salt, and cooked sweet potatoes until smooth (or mash the ingredients in a large bowl by hand as you please).

Add the cooked onions and spices to the sweet potato mixture in a big mixing bowl.

A broad baking dish should be lightly oiled.

Fill each tortilla with around 2/3 to 3/4 cup of the filling, roll it up, and put it seam side down in the baking dish.

Bake for 30 minutes, or until piping hot, covered tightly with foil.

Serve with salsa on top.

PERFECT CAULIFLOWER PIZZA CRUST

INGREDIENTS

- 4 cups raw cauliflower, riced or 1 medium cauliflower head
- 1 egg, beaten
- 1 cup chevre cheese or 1 cup other soft cheese
- 1 teaspoon dried oregano
- 1 pinch salt

DIRECTIONS

Preheat the oven to 400 degrees Fahrenheit.

To make the cauliflower rice, pulse batches of raw cauliflower florets in a food processor until they have a rice-like texture.

Bring a big pot of water to a boil with about an inch of water in it. Cook for about 4-5 minutes after adding the "rice" and covering it. Drain into a strainer with a fine mesh.

THE SECRET: Once the rice has been strained, move it to a clean, thin dishtowel. SQUEEZE all the extra moisture out of the steamed rice by wrapping it in a dishtowel, twisting it up. It's incredible how much extra liquid would be released, resulting in a clean, dry pizza crust.

Combine the strained rice, beaten egg, goat cheese, and spices in a wide mixing bowl. (Don't be shy about using your hands! You want it to be thoroughly mixed.) It won't be like any other pizza dough you've made before, but don't worry: it'll hold together!

Line a baking sheet with parchment paper and place the dough on it. (It must be lined with parchment paper or else it would stick.) Keep the dough about 3/8" thick, and if you like, raise the edges for a "crust" effect.

Preheat oven to 400°F and bake for 35-40 minutes. When finished, the crust should be strong and golden brown.

Now is the time to add all of your favourite toppings, including sauce, cheese, and any other ingredients you need. Return the pizza to the oven at 400°F for another 5-10 minutes, or until the cheese is hot and bubbly.

SHEET PAN CHICKEN AND BRUSSEL SPROUTS

INGREDIENTS

- 4 skin on chicken thighs
- 1 1/2 cups Brussels sprouts, halved
- 4 carrots, cut on the bias
- 3 tablespoons olive oil
- 1 teaspoon herbes de provence

DIRECTIONS

Preheat the oven to 400 degrees Fahrenheit.

Toss cut vegetables with 1 1/2 tbsp olive oil, 12 tsp herbs, and salt and pepper in a dish. Rub the vegetables all over.

Arrange the vegetables on a sheet tray.

In the same dish, position the chicken thighs. Drizzle with 1/12 tablespoons olive oil, 12 tablespoons herbs, and season with salt and pepper. Rub the chicken all over.

Place the chicken in the tub.

Roast the chicken for 30-35 minutes, or until it is completely cooked.

Switch the oven to broil and cook for a minute or two if you prefer a crispier vegetable or chicken skin. If you don't keep an eye on it, it will burn.

BROCCOLI DAL CURRY

INGREDIENTS

- 4 tablespoons butter or 4 tablespoons ghee
- 2 medium onions, chopped
- 1 teaspoon chili powder
- 1 1/2 teaspoons black pepper
- 2 teaspoons cumin
- 1 teaspoon ground coriander
- 2 teaspoons turmeric
- 1 cup red lentil
- 1 lemon, juice of
- 3 cups chicken broth
- 2 medium broccoli, chopped
- 1/2 cup dried coconut (optional)
- 1 tablespoon flour
- 1 teaspoon salt
- 1 cup cashews, coarsely chopped (optional)

DIRECTIONS

Melt the butter in a saucepan and brown the onions.

Chili powder, pepper, cumin, coriander, and turmeric are all good additions.

1 minute of stirring and cooking

Add the lentils, lemon juice, broth, and, if using, the coconut.

Bring to a boil, then reduce to a low heat and cook for 45-55 minutes (if mixture is too thick, you may need to add a little hot water).

7 minutes of steaming broccoli

Set aside broccoli after submerging it in cold water.

Remove 1/3 cup of the lentil mixture's liquid.

To make a smooth paste, mix in the flour.

Return to the pan and stir in the broccoli, salt, and nuts, if desired.

Cook for 5 minutes on low heat.

Over Basmati rice, serve.

BAKED MAHI MAHI

INGREDIENTS

- 2 lbs mahi mahi (4 fillets)
- 1 lemon, juiced
- 1/4 teaspoon garlic salt
- 1/4 teaspoon ground black pepper
- 1 cup mayonnaise
- 1/4 cup white onion, finely chopped
- breadcrumbs

DIRECTIONS

Preheat the oven to 425 degrees Fahrenheit.

Place the fish in a baking dish after rinsing it. Squeeze lemon juice over the fish, then season with salt and pepper.

Spread mayonnaise and chopped onions on the trout. Bake for 25 minutes at 425°F with breadcrumbs on top.

CAJUN POTATO, PRAWN/SHRIMP AND AVOCADO SALAD

INGREDIENTS

- 300g new potatoes (small baby or chats 10 oz halved)
- 1tablespoon olive oil
- 250 g king prawns (8 oz, cooked and peeled)
- 1 garlic clove (minced)
- 2 spring onions (finely sliced)
- 2 teaspoons cajun seasoning
- 1 avocado (peeled, stoned and diced)
- 1 cup alfalfa sprout
- salt (to boil potatoes)

DIRECTIONS

Cook the potatoes for 10 to 15 minutes, or until tender, in a large saucepan of lightly salted boiling water. Drain well.

In a wok or big nonstick frying pan/skillet, heat the oil.

Stir in the prawns, garlic, spring onions, and Cajun seasoning until the prawns are sweet, around 2 to 3 minutes.

Cook for another minute after adding the potatoes.

Transfer to serving dishes and garnish with avocado and alfalfa sprouts until serving.

WARM ROASTED VEGETABLE FARRO SALAD

INGREDIENTS

- 1/2 medium sized eggplant, peel on and large diced
- 1 tablespoon kosher salt or 1 tablespoon sea salt
- 1 cup cherry tomatoes, washed and left whole
- 1 medium sized zucchini, peel on and large diced
- 6 white button mushrooms, quartered
- 6 garlic cloves, peeled, trimmed and sliced
- 1/2 medium sized red onion, peeled and cut into wedges
- 1 tablespoon olive oil
- 1 cup cracked farro
- 2 cups almond milk (Almond Breeze)
- 1 teaspoon tbsp olive oil (15 mL)
- 1 tablespoon olive oil
- 1 tablespoon balsamic vinegar
- 3 sprigs fresh cilantro
- 1/2 teaspoon salt
- 1/2 teaspoon pepper

DIRECTIONS

Strat with preheat the oven to 400 degrees Fahrenheit (200 degrees Celsius).

Salt the eggplant slices generously on all sides in a wide flat pan or baking sheet, toss to coat evenly, and set aside for 30 minutes to release excess moisture and bitterness.

Toss the eggplant into a big mixing bowl after draining and rinsing it. Combine the tomatoes, zucchini, mushrooms, garlic, and onions in a large mixing bowl. Drizzle olive oil over the vegetables and season with salt and pepper, tossing to coat. Transfer the vegetables to a tin foil-lined ovenproof tray.

Roast the vegetables for 20 to 25 minutes, or until they are smooth, caramelised, and fork tender. To keep the vegetables from sticking to the plate, stir or flip them after 10–15 minutes of roasting. Place the pan on a cooling rack after removing it from the oven.

Meanwhile, drain the farro in a colander over the sink after rinsing it with water. In a 3-quart (3L) saucepot, combine the farro and Almond Breeze. Add a pinch of salt and a drizzle of olive oil to taste. To stop spilling, bring the liquid to a boil over medium-high heat and then reduce to a low simmer.

Cook the farro for 20 minutes with the lid cocked to one side to allow steam to escape. Remove the pot from the heat but keep it on the stovetop and close the lid. Steam for an additional 5 minutes in the pot, or until the farro is soft but slightly chewy in the middle. After removing the lid, fluff with a fork.

Combine the cooked farro and vegetables in a large serving dish and gently toss to combine when ready to serve. Combine the olive oil and balsamic vinegar in a mixing bowl and drizzle over the farro salad. Toss to coat and season to taste with salt and pepper. Serve with a squeeze of lemon and fresh cilantro on top. Heat the dish before serving.

TRAIL MIX

INGREDIENTS

- 1 cup almonds (raw)
- 1 cup sunflower seeds (raw)
- 1 cup raisins
- 1/2 cup dried apricot (unsulphured, chopped)
- 1/4 cup flaked coconut (optional)
- 1/4 cup chocolate (optional) or 1/4 cup carob chips (optional)

DIRECTIONS

Combine all ingredients in a big container, cover, and shake!

Keep the jar airtight. Refrigerate or freeze to preserve the essential fatty acid properties.

PERFECT HARD BOILED EGGS

INGREDIENTS

- 6 large eggs
- water

DIRECTIONS

In a medium saucepan, crack the eggs. 1" above the chickens, cover with water. Place on high heat on the stovetop.

Get the water to a boil. Remove from heat and cover immediately. Allow for 18-20 minutes of resting time.

Keeping the pot on a slant, pour cold tap water into the pot, allowing the hot water to escape. Allow eggs to sit in cold water for 1-2 minutes before peeling.

NOTE: Peel the eggs under cold running water with a colander underneath to catch the shells (no garbage disposal/shells for gardening method). For egg salad, I used paper towels to absorb excess moisture, but peeled eggs can also be put in a bowl of cold water, covered, and refrigerated for up to 4-5 days.

BERRY CRISP

INGREDIENTS

FRUIT

- 1 (16 ounce) bag cherries or (16 ounce) bag blueberries
- 1 (7/8 ounce) box jello sugar-free vanilla pudding mix, cook and serve
- 1 teaspoon cinnamon
- 1/2 teaspoon nutmeg
- 1/4 cup nonfat milk

CRISP

- 1 1/2 cups old fashioned oats 1/2
- cup Splenda sugar substitute 8 ounces plain fat-free yogurt
- 1 teaspoon almond extract

DIRECTIONS

An 8X8 baking pan should be sprayed.

In a pan, combine the fruit ingredients and stir well.

Crisp mix should be combined in a separate tub.

To make a top crust, spread this mixture over the berry mixture.

Preheat oven to 350°F and bake for 40-45 minutes, or until topping is crunchy.

SAUERKRAUT SALAD

INGREDIENTS

- 1 (1 lb) can sauerkraut, drained but not rinsed
- 1 cup celery, chopped fine
- 1⁄2 cup green pepper, chopped fine
- 2 tablespoons onions, chopped fine
- 1⁄2 teaspoon salt
- 1⁄2 teaspoon pepper
- 3⁄4 cup sugar
- 1⁄3 cup salad oil
- 1⁄3 cup cider (I use white) or 1/3 cup white vinegar (I use white)

DIRECTIONS

Combine chopped vegetables and sauerkraut in a mixing bowl.

Heat the sugar, oil, vinegar, salt, and pepper in a small saucepan over low heat until the sugar has dissolved.

Allow to cool before pouring over the vegetables.

Allow to chill overnight.

VEGAN COCONUT KEFIR BANANA MUFFINS

INGREDIENTS

- 2 cups all-purpose flour
- 1 cup granulated sugar
- 1 cup unsweetened dried shredded coconut
- 2 teaspoons baking soda
- 1 teaspoon baking powder
- 1/2 teaspoon salt
- 2 ripe bananas, mashed
- 1 1/2 cups pc dairy-free kefir probiotic fermented coconut milk
- 1/4 cup cold-pressed liquid coconut oil
- 1 teaspoon vanilla extract

DIRECTIONS

1. Start with preheat the oven to 350 degrees Fahrenheit (180 degrees Celsius). Using cooking spray, spray a 12-count muffin tin. Remove from the equation.

2. In a big mixing bowl, combine flour, sugar, coconut, baking soda, baking powder, and salt. Remove from the equation.

3. In a separate large mixing bowl, combine the bananas, kefir, coconut oil, and vanilla. Add to flour mixture and whisk until there are no white streaks left.

4. Divide the batter evenly among the muffin tin wells. Bake for about 30 minutes, or until the tops are golden and a toothpick inserted in the centre comes out clean. Allow 15 minutes for cooling in the muffin pan.

Allow muffins to cool fully on a wire rack before transferring to an airtight container or resealable freezer bag and freezing for up to one month. Cover the muffins individually in plastic wrap or foil before putting them in the tub or bag to protect them from freezer burn. Muffins can be thawed overnight in the fridge or warmed in the microwave for 20 to 30 seconds straight from frozen.

VEGAN LENTIL BURGERS

INGREDIENTS

- 1 cup dry lentils, well rinsed
- 2 1/2 cups water
- 1/2 teaspoon salt
- 1 tablespoon olive oil
- 1/2 medium onion, diced
- 1 carrot, diced
- 1 teaspoon pepper
- 1 tablespoon soy sauce
- 3/4 cup rolled oats, finely ground
- 3/4 cup breadcrumbs

DIRECTIONS

Lentils should be cooked for 45 minutes in salted water. The lentils will be soft and much of the liquid will have evaporated.

In a small amount of oil, fry the onions and carrots until tender, around 5 minutes.

Combine the cooked ingredients, pepper, soy sauce, oats, and bread crumbs in a mixing bowl.

Shape the mixture into patties while it is still warm; it will make 8-10 burgers.

After that, the burgers can be shallow fried for 1-2 minutes on each side or baked for 15 minutes at 200°C.

BLACK BEAN SOUP

INGREDIENTS

- 3 tablespoons olive oil
- 1 medium onion, chopped
- 1 tablespoon ground cumin
- 2 -3 cloves garlic
- 2 (14 1/2 ounce) cans black beans
- 2 cups chicken broth or 2 cups vegetable broth
- salt and pepper
- 1 small red onion, chopped fine
- 1/4 cup cilantro, coarsely chopped or finely chopped (whatever you prefer)

DIRECTIONS

In a normal pan, sauté the onion in olive oil.

Cumin should be added until the onion has become translucent.

Cook for 30 seconds before adding the garlic and continuing to cook for another 30 to 60 seconds.

2 cups vegetable broth and 1 can black beans

Bring to a low heat and cook, stirring occasionally.

Switch the heat off.

Blend the ingredients in the pot with a hand blender or move to a blender.

Bring the second can of beans, as well as the blended ingredients, to a simmer in the oven.

For garnish, serve the soup with bowls of red onion and cilantro.

In the pot, I also throw in some cilantro.

This recipe can be doubled or frozen.

BAKED POTATO

INGREDIENTS

- 1 large russet potato
- canola oil
- kosher salt

DIRECTIONS

Preheat the oven to 350°F and arrange the racks in the upper and lower thirds.

Wash the potato (or potatoes) vigorously under cold running water with a stiff brush.

Dry the spud, then poke 8 to 12 deep holes all over it with a standard fork to allow moisture to escape during cooking.

Place in a bowl with a thin coating of oil.

Season with kosher salt and put directly on the oven's middle rack.

CAULIFLOWER POPCORN - ROASTED CAULIFLOWER

INGREDIENTS

- 1 head cauliflower or 1 head equal amount of pre-cut commercially prepped cauliflower
- 4 tablespoons olive oil
- 1 teaspoon salt, to taste

DIRECTIONS

Preheat the oven to 425 degrees Fahrenheit.

Trim the cauliflower head, discarding the heart and thick stems; cut the florets into ping-pong-ball-sized pieces.

Whisk together the olive oil and salt in a big mixing bowl, then add the cauliflower pieces and toss well.

Spread the cauliflower parts on a baking sheet lined with parchment paper for easy cleanup (you can skip this if you don't have any), then roast for 1 hour, turning 3 or 4 times until the majority of the pieces are golden brown.

The more caramelization happens and the sweeter the cauliflower parts taste, the browner they become.

Serve right away and enjoy!

ROASTED BROCCOLI WITH TOASTED PINE NUTS LEMON & GARLIC

INGREDIENTS

- 1 lb broccoli floret
- 2 tablespoons olive oil
- salt & freshly ground black pepper
- 2 tablespoons unsalted butter
- 1 teaspoon garlic, minced
- 1/2 teaspoon lemon zest, grated
- 1 -2 tablespoon fresh lemon juice
- 2 tablespoons pine nuts, toasted

DIRECTIONS

Preheat the oven to 500 degrees Fahrenheit.

Toss the broccoli with the oil and salt and pepper to taste in a big mixing bowl.

Roast the florets in a single layer on a baking sheet for 12 minutes, or until only tender, turning once.

Meanwhile, melt the butter in a small saucepan over medium heat.

Heat the garlic and lemon zest for about 1 minute, stirring constantly.

Allow for a brief cooling period before adding the lemon juice.

Place the broccoli in a serving bowl and toss with the lemon butter to cover.

Sprinkle the toasted pine nuts on top.

SHREDDED BRUSSELS SPROUTS WITH BACON AND ONIONS

INGREDIENTS

- 2 slices bacon
- 1 small yellow onion, thinly sliced
- 1/4 teaspoon salt (or to taste)
- 3/4 cup water
- 1 teaspoon Dijon mustard
- 1 lb Brussels sprout, trimmed, halved and very thinly sliced
- 1 tablespoon cider vinegar

DIRECTIONS

Cook bacon until crisp in a large skillet over medium heat (5–7 minutes); drain on paper towels, then crumble.

Toss the onion and salt into the drippings in the pan and cook, stirring frequently, until tender and browned (about 3 minutes).

Scrape up any browned bits with water and mustard, then add Brussels sprouts and cook, stirring frequently, until tender (4 to 6 minutes).

Add the vinegar and crumbled bacon on top.

SUPPER CLUB TILAPIA PARMESAN

INGREDIENTS

- 2 lbs tilapia fillets (orange roughy, cod or red snapper can be substituted)
- 2 tablespoons lemon juice
- 1/2 cup grated parmesan cheese
- 4 tablespoons butter, room temperature
- 3 tablespoons mayonnaise
- 3 tablespoons finely chopped green onions
- 1/4 teaspoon seasoning salt (I like Old Bay seasoning here)
- 1/4 teaspoon dried basil
- black pepper
- 1 dash hot pepper sauce

DIRECTIONS

Preheat the oven to 350 degrees Fahrenheit.

Arrange the fillets in a single layer in a buttered 13-by-9-inch baking dish or jellyroll tray.

Fillets should not be stacked.

Apply some juice to the tip.

Combine the cheese, butter, mayonnaise, onions, and seasonings in a mixing bowl.

With a fork, thoroughly combine the ingredients.

Bake the fish for 10 to 20 minutes in a preheated oven, or until it begins to flake.

Spread the cheese mixture on top and bake for 5 minutes, or until golden brown.

The length of time it takes to bake the fish will be determined by its thickness.

Make sure the fish doesn't overcook by keeping an eye on it.

This recipe serves 4 people.

This fish can also be cooked in the broiler.

3–4 minutes under the broiler, or until almost done.

Broil for another 2 to 3 minutes, or until cheese is browned.

MEDITERRANEAN CHICKEN BREASTS WITH AVOCADO TAPENADE

INGREDIENTS

- 4 boneless skinless chicken breast halves
- 1 tablespoon grated lemon peel
- 5 tablespoons fresh lemon juice, divided
- 2 tablespoons olive oil, divided
- 1 teaspoon olive oil, divided
- 1 garlic clove, finely chopped
- 1/2 teaspoon salt
- 1/4 teaspoon ground black pepper
- 2 garlic cloves, roasted and mashed
- 1/2 teaspoon sea salt
- 1/4 teaspoon fresh ground pepper
- 1 medium tomatoes, seeded and finely chopped
- 1/4 cup small green pimento stuffed olive, thinly sliced
- 3 tablespoons capers, rinsed
- 2 tablespoons fresh basil leaves, finely sliced
- 1 large Hass avocado, ripe, finely chopped

DIRECTIONS

In a sealable plastic bag, combine the chicken, lemon peel, 2 tablespoons lemon juice, 2 tablespoons olive oil, garlic, salt, and pepper.

Refrigerate for 30 minutes after sealing the container.

Combine the remaining 3 tablespoons lemon juice, roasted garlic, 1/2 teaspoon olive oil, sea salt, and freshly ground pepper in a mixing bowl. Set aside the onion, green olives, capers, basil, and avocado.

Remove the chicken from the bag and toss out the marinade. Grill for 4 to 5 minutes per side over medium-hot coals, or until desired degree of doneness is reached.

Avocado Tapenade is a great addition to this dish.

VEGAN FRIED 'FISH' TACOS

INGREDIENTS

- 14 ounces silken tofu
- 2 cups panko breadcrumbs
- 1/2 cup plain flour
- 1/2 teaspoon salt
- 1 teaspoon smoked paprika
- 1/2 teaspoon cayenne pepper
- 1 teaspoon ground cumin
- 1/2 cup non-dairy milk
- vegetable oil, for frying
- 1/4 head cabbage, finely shredded
- 1 ripe avocado
- 8 small tortillas
- vegan mayonnaise, to serve
- pickled onion
- 1 red onion, peeled, finely sliced
- 1/4 cup apple cider vinegar
- 1 tablespoon sugar
- 1 teaspoon salt

DIRECTIONS

To extract excess moisture, pat the tofu with a few pieces of kitchen paper. Split the tofu into rough 1-inch pieces with a knife – I prefer them to be imperfect, rather than cubes, so they look better!

Combine the breadcrumbs in a big shallow bowl.

In a separate large shallow cup, combine the flour, salt, smoked paprika, cayenne, and cumin.

In a third big shallow tub, pour the milk.

Toss the tofu chunks in the flour, then the milk, then the breadcrumbs, and place them on a baking sheet.

Fill a deep frying pan with vegetable oil to a depth of 1/2 inch. Place over a medium heat and allow the oil to heat up – if a breadcrumb begins to bubble and brown, the oil is ready. Fry chunks of breaded tofu until golden underneath, then flip and finish cooking until golden all over. To drain, place on a baking sheet lined with kitchen paper. Rep with the rest of the tofu.

Pickled Onion

In a small pot, heat the apple cider vinegar, salt, and sugar until steaming. Pour the hot vinegar over the finely sliced red onion in a bowl or pot. Allow it to soften and turn pink for at least 30 minutes.

Serve the spicy fried tofu with pickled onion, vegan mayo, avocado, and shredded cabbage in warmed tortillas (I warm mine over a lit gas ring on my stove).

COBB SALAD WITH BROWN DERBY DRESSING

INGREDIENTS

- 1/2 head iceberg lettuce
- 1/2 bunch watercress
- 1 bunch chicory lettuce
- 1/2 head romaine lettuce
- 2 medium tomatoes, skinned and seeded
- 1/2 lb smoked turkey breast
- 6 slices crisp bacon
- 1 avocado, sliced in half,seeded and peeled
- 3 hardboiled egg
- 2 tablespoons chives, chopped fine
- 1/2 cup blue cheese, crumbled

DRESSING

- 2 tablespoons water
- 1/8 teaspoon sugar
- 3/4 teaspoon kosher salt
- 1/2 teaspoon Worcestershire sauce
- 2 tablespoons balsamic vinegar (or red wine vinegar)
- 1 tablespoon fresh lemon juice
- 1/2 teaspoon fresh ground black pepper
- 1/8 teaspoon Dijon mustard

- 2 tablespoons olive oil
- 2 cloves garlic, minced very fine

DIRECTIONS

Finely chop all of the greens (almost minced).

In a chilled salad bowl, arrange in rows.

Cut the tomatoes in half, remove the seeds, and chop finely.

The ham, avocado, eggs, and bacon should all be finely diced.

Arrange all of the ingredients in rows around the lettuces, including the blue cheese.

Lastly, add the chives.

Present in this manner at the table, then toss with the dressing just before serving in chilled salad bowls.

Serve with a side of freshly baked French bread.

TO MAKE THE DRESSING: In a blender, combine all of the ingredients, except the olive oil, and blend until smooth.

Slowly drizzle in the oil when the unit is working, and thoroughly blend.

Keep refrigerated until ready to use.

***NOTE:** Keep this dish chilled and eat it, as chilled as possible.

VEGGIE PACKED CHEESY CHICKEN SALAD (REDUCED FAT)

INGREDIENTS

- 1 cup cooked boneless skinless chicken breast, cubed
- 1/4 cup celery, finely chopped
- 1/4 cup carrot, shaved into ribbons
- 1/2 cup Baby Spinach, roughly chopped
- 2 1/2 tablespoons fat-free mayonnaise
- 2 tablespoons nonfat sour cream
- 1/8 teaspoon dried parsley
- 2 teaspoons Dijon mustard
- 1/4 cup reduced-fat sharp cheddar cheese, shredded

DIRECTIONS

In a mixing bowl, combine all ingredients and coat thoroughly with the mayonnaise mixture.

Refrigerate for at least 30 minutes, but it's better if you do it the night before.

Enjoy!

AVOCADO QUESADILLAS

INGREDIENTS

- 2 vine-ripe tomatoes, seeded and chopped into 1/4 inch pieces
- 1 ripe avocado, peeled, pitted, and chopped into 1/4 inch pieces
- 1 tablespoon chopped red onion
- 2 teaspoons fresh lemon juice
- 1/4 teaspoon Tabasco sauce
- salt and pepper
- 1/4 cup sour cream
- 3 tablespoons chopped fresh coriander
- 24 inches flour tortillas
- 1/2 teaspoon vegetable oil
- 1 1/3 cups shredded monterey jack cheese

DIRECTIONS

Combine the tomatoes, avocado, onion, lemon juice, and Tabasco in a small bowl.

Season with salt and pepper to taste.

Mix sour cream, coriander, salt, and pepper to taste in a separate small cup.

Brush the tops of the tortillas with oil and place them on a baking sheet.

2 to 4 inches from the sun, broil tortillas until pale golden.

Sprinkle cheese uniformly over tortillas and broil until melted.

To make 2 quesadillas, spread avocado mixture evenly over 2 tortillas and cover each with 1 of the remaining tortillas, cheese side down.

Break the quesadillas into four wedges on a cutting board.

Serve warm with a dollop of sour cream mixture on top of each wedge.

GRILLED LEMON SALMON

INGREDIENTS

- 2 teaspoons fresh dill
- 1/2 teaspoon pepper
- 1/2 teaspoon salt
- 1/2 teaspoon garlic powder
- 1 1/2 lbs salmon fillets
- 1/4 cup packed brown sugar
- 1 chicken bouillon cube, mixed with
- 3 tablespoons water
- 3 tablespoons oil
- 3 tablespoons soy sauce
- 4 tablespoons finely chopped green onions
- 1 lemon, thinly sliced
- 2 slices onions, seperated into rings

DIRECTIONS

Season the salmon with dill, pepper, salt, and garlic powder.

Fill a shallow glass pan halfway with water.

Combine the sugar, chicken broth, oil, soy sauce, and green onions in a mixing bowl.

Pour the sauce over the salmon.

Cover and chill for 1 hour, turning halfway through.

Drain and toss out the marinade.

Place lemon and onion on top of grill on medium heat.

Cook for 15 minutes, or until fish is thoroughly cooked.

For the most part, intermittent fasting is healthy. Intermittent fasting, however, has been shown in research to have some mild side effects. Furthermore, it is not the only option for anyone.

HUNGER AND CRAVINGS

Hunger is one of the most common side effects of intermittent fasting, which comes as no surprise. You can feel increased hunger if you minimize your calorie intake or go long stretches without eating.

Some 112 people were randomly allocated to an intermittent energy restriction category in a survey. For a year, they ate 400 or 600 calories on two nonconsecutive days per week. These individuals reported feeling hungrier than those who followed a low-calorie diet with constant calorie restriction.

According to studies, hunger is a common symptom people encounter within the first few days of a fasting regimen. In a 2020 survey, 1,422 people took part in fasting regimens that lasted 4–21 days. Only within the first few days of the regimens did they experience hunger symptoms.

As a result, hunger symptoms can fade as your body adjusts to normal fasting periods.

HEADACHES AND LIGHTHEADEDNESS

Intermittent fasting is also associated with headaches. They usually happen in the first few days of a fasting regimen. In a study published in 2020, researchers looked at 18 studies involving people who practiced intermittent fasting. Any participants in the four studies who reported side effects said they had moderate headaches.

Researchers also discovered that "fasting headaches" are normally located in the frontal area of the brain, with pain that is mild to moderate in severity. Furthermore, people who suffer from headaches often are more likely to suffer from headaches when fasting than those who do not.

Low blood sugar and caffeine withdrawal, according to research, can lead to headaches during intermittent fasting.

DIGESTIVE ISSUES

If you do intermittent fasting, you can experience digestive problems such as constipation, diarrhea, nausea, and bloating.

The reduction in food intake that certain intermittent fasting regimens entails can have a detrimental impact on your digestion, resulting in constipation and other unpleasant side effects. Additionally, dietary changes associated with intermittent fasting programs can result in bloating and diarrhea.

Constipation may be exacerbated by dehydration, another popular side effect of intermittent fasting. As a result, it's important to remain well hydrated while fasting intermittently. Constipation can be avoided by eating nutrient-dense, fiber-rich foods.

IRRITABILITY AND OTHER MOOD CHANGES

When people practice intermittent fasting, they can experience irritability and other mood swings. When your blood sugar levels are poor, you can become irritable.

Hypoglycemia, or low blood sugar, can occur during periods of calorie restriction or fasting. Irritability, anxiety, and low focus are all possible outcomes.

A 2016 study of 52 women found that during an 18-hour fasting cycle, participants were substantially more irritable than during a non-fasting period.

Interestingly, the researchers discovered that, although the women were irritable at the end of the fasting era, they also felt a greater sense of accomplishment, dignity, and self-control than they did at the beginning.

FATIGUE AND LOW ENERGY

Some people who practice different forms of intermittent fasting feel exhaustion and low energy levels, according to studies.

Intermittent fasting can make you feel exhausted and weak due to low blood sugar. In addition, intermittent fasting can cause sleep disturbances in some people, resulting in fatigue during the day.

Intermittent fasting, on the other hand, has been shown in some studies to reduce fatigue, especially as your body adapts to daily fasting periods.

BAD BREATH

Bad breath is an unwanted side effect that some people experience when they fast intermittently. Lack of salivary flow and an increase in acetone in the breath trigger this. Fasting allows the body to burn fat as a source of energy. Since acetone is a waste product of fat metabolism, it accumulates in your blood and breath when you fast. Dehydration, which is a sign of intermittent fasting, may also trigger dry mouth, which can lead to bad breath.

SLEEP DISTURBANCES

According to some studies, sleep disturbances, such as inability to fall or remain asleep, are one of the most common side effects of intermittent fasting. In a 2020 survey, 1,422 people took part in fasting regimens that lasted 4–21 days. Fasting caused sleep disturbances in 15% of the participants, according to the report. This was mentioned more often than other side effects.

Since your body excretes large quantities of salt and water through the urine, fatigue can be more normal in the early days of an intermittent fasting regimen. Dehydration and low salt levels can result as a result of this.

MALNUTRITION

Intermittent fasting, if performed incorrectly, will result in malnutrition. Malnutrition can occur when an individual fasts for long periods of time and does not replenish their body with enough nutrients. The same can be said for unplanned, long-term energy restriction diets.

On different forms of intermittent fasting systems, people are usually able to fulfil their calorie and nutrient requirements.

However, if you don't properly schedule or execute the fasting regimen for a long period of time, or if you intentionally limit calories to an excessive amount, you risk malnutrition and other health problems.

That's why, when fasting intermittently, it's important to eat a well-balanced, healthy diet. Make sure you're not restricting your calorie consumption too much.

A healthcare professional who is familiar with intermittent fasting will assist you in developing a healthy plan that offers the right number of calories and nutrients for you.

Intermittent fasting can be a good idea for some people, but it isn't suitable or healthy for others. Intermittent fasting has the potential to cause dangerous side effects in certain people.

Intermittent fasting is usually advised against by healthcare practitioners for the following people:

- Women who are pregnant or who are breast-feeding/chest-feeding small children or teenagers
- Elderly people who are experiencing fatigue
- Immunocompromised individuals
- Women who are now or have previously struggled with eating disorders
- Alzheimer's patients
- Women who have had a traumatic brain injury or have suffered from post-concussive syndrome

Furthermore, if you experience long-term side effects from intermittent fasting, it may be an indication that it isn't working for you. The following are examples of possible side effects:

- nausea
- headaches
- irritability
- faintness
- fatigue
- extreme hunger

If you're unhappy with intermittent fasting, don't keep doing it.

Even though fasting has been linked to health benefits, there are several other ways to improve your health that do not require fasting.

Following a well-balanced and healthy diet, getting enough sleep, engaging in daily physical activity, and managing stress are all important for better health.

CONCLUSION

Anyone does not need to practice intermittent fasting. It's only one of the lifestyle changes that will help you live a healthier life. The most important things to remember are to keep eating real food, exercising, and sleeping sufficiently. If you don't like the concept of fasting, you can easily disregard this article and continue doing what you want.

There is no such thing as a one-size-fits-all solution when it comes to nutrition. The safest diet for you is one that you can maintain over time. Dedicated people benefit from intermittent fasting, and many others do not. Only by trying it out can you figure out which group you belong to.

If you enjoy fasting and believe it is a sustainable way of eating, it can be a very useful method for losing weight and improving your health.

Intermittent fasting has been linked to a variety of health benefits, including reduced heart problems risk factors, weight loss, better blood sugar regulation, and more. Intermittent fasting is usually thought to be harmless, but studies have shown that it can cause hunger, constipation, irritability, headaches, and bad breath.

In addition, some healthcare practitioners warn against intermittent fasting. People who are pregnant or breastfeeding as well as those who have eating disorders, fall into this category.

If you're thinking of trying intermittent fasting, talk to your doctor first to make sure it's a safe and healthy option for you.